Moving Beyond The Covid-19 Lies Together:

Renewing Hope For Humanity Through Untold Truth About The Pandemic Inspired by Dr. Bryan Ardis

Mark B. Williams

All rights reserved. No part of this publication may be reproduced, distributed, or transmitted in any form or by any means, including photocopying, recording, or other electronic or mechanical methods, without the prior written permission of the publisher, except in the case of brief quotations embodied in critical reviews and certain other noncommercial uses permitted by copyright law.

Copyright ©Mark B. Williams 2025

Table Of Contents:

Did A Bat Really Cough And Make The Entire World Sick :

Facts About Remdesivir

The COVID Heart

Arizona University:

Issue with Clotting:

Could Snakes Be The Original Source?

Shereen's story: my lengthy COVID experience

Long COVID: What Is It?

Did A Bat Really Cough And Make The Entire World Sick :

In southern China, a nameless parasite coexisted peacefully with horseshoe bats for thousands of years. The bats were so advanced that they were unaware of it and continued their nighttime travels without any problems. The parasite, an ancestor of the coronavirus SARS-CoV-2, had a chance to spread its domain one day. The pangolin, also known as the scaly anteater, is an endangered species that is often trafficked and sold in secret at live animal markets throughout China and Southeast Asia. Or not. Uncertainty surrounds the genetic route. However, the virus had to undergo a significant mutation in order to live in a new species, whatever it was. It may have even grabbed a piece of another coronavirus strain that was already present in its new host and changed into a hybrid—a more powerful and superior form of itself, a pathogenic Everyman that could survive in a variety of animals. Our species was discovered by the coronavirus more recently. A tired traveler could have scratched his nose, wiped his eyes, or inadvertently and frantically chewed his fingernails. One little, undetectable viral glob. A single human face. We are now fighting a worldwide epidemic.

From around 213 thousand on March 19 to 467 thousand on March 26, the number of confirmed patients worldwide (those with a positive lab test for COVID-19, the illness caused by SARS-CoV-2) quadrupled in only seven days. There have been over 21,000 fatalities. As of March 26th, the United States has more confirmed cases than any other nation in the world, with over 80,000 cases. These figures represent a small portion of the actual, unknowable total in this nation and globally, and they will continue to rise. According to a recent research by scientists that was published earlier this month in the journal Science, there are probably five to ten additional community members who are infected but have not been identified for every verified case. This is probably going to stay the same. One of the study's authors, Jeffrey Shaman, a professor of environmental-health sciences at Columbia University, said that the testing was "far from adequate." Doctors' comments from emergency rooms have begun going viral on social media. One, from Bergamo, north of Milan, doctor Daniele Macchini, called the situation a "tsunami that has overwhelmed us."

After the 2003 Severe Acute Respiratory Syndrome (SARS) epidemic, researchers first learned that coronaviruses are bat-borne. One member of a research team that searched for the source in China's Guangdong Province, where concurrent SARS outbreaks had occurred, was Jonathan Epstein, an epidemiologist at the EcoHealth Alliance in New York who specializes in zoonotic viruses, or viruses that can spread from animals to humans. This suggests that there were multiple spillovers from animals to humans. Since palm civets, a mongoose-like animal that is often consumed in areas of China, were sold at markets linked to the SARS epidemic and tested positive for the virus, health authorities first thought they were to blame. However, civets grown in other parts of Guangdong did not have any antibodies against the virus, suggesting that the market animals were only a highly contagious intermediate host. Bats, which are common in the rural, agricultural hills of the region and were, at the time, being sold from cages at Guangdong's wet markets, were suspected by Epstein and others of serving as the coronavirus's natural reservoir.

While traveling across the countryside, the researchers set up field laboratories within caves made of limestone and collected swabs from hundreds of bats throughout the night. Four species of horseshoe bats carrying coronaviruses related to SARS were found by Epstein's team after months of research; one of these species had a coronavirus that was more than 90% genetically identical. "They were discovered in every area where SARS clusters were occurring," he said.

Researchers ultimately discovered the direct coronavirus antecedent to SARS after years of more bat monitoring. They also discovered hundreds of other coronaviruses spreading among some of the fourteen hundred bat species that inhabit six continents. It turns out that coronaviruses and other virus families have co-evolved with bats for as long as human civilization has existed, and maybe much longer. As the coronavirus family expands, many strains co-infect individual bats at the same time, transforming their tiny bodies into virus blenders that produce new strains of all kinds, some more potent than others. Scientists have connected the unique ability of bats to fly among mammals to this mechanism, which occurs without making the bats ill. Their immune systems have developed a better method to mend damaged cells and fend off infections without causing further inflammation as a result of the feat's harsh toll. However, these viruses may cause serious, perhaps fatal illness when they infect a new species, such as humans, civets, or pangolins.

Shi Zheng-Li, Epstein's principal Chinese colleague, sequenced a bat coronavirus in 2013 and determined in January that it shared 96% of its genome with SARS-CoV-2. Although the two viruses share an ancestor that is between thirty and fifty years old, the lack of a perfect match indicates that more mutation occurred in other bat colonies before spreading to an intermediate host. Many of the 41 severe instances of pneumonia that were first reported in Wuhan in December were linked to a wet market that had an infamous animal department. Cages are piled high with animals—ferret-badgers on top of civets and rabbits on top of one other. Epstein said, "That's just a gravitational exchange of viruses and fecal matter." Chinese officials said that they tested animals at the market, and all of the results were negative. However, they did not identify which animals were examined, which is important information for Epstein's investigative work. The virus was eventually discovered by authorities in samples collected from the market's gutters and tables. However, Epstein noted that "it raised the question of, well, perhaps those forty-one weren't the first cases" since not all of the first patients were linked to the market or to one other.

It seems probable that the virus was circulating among humans before December because genomic analyses of SARS-CoV-2 show a single spillover event, which means the virus only moved from an animal to a human once. The transmission chain could never be known until further details about the animals in the Wuhan market are made public. However, there are a lot of options. The virus may have entered the market by a wildlife trafficker or a bat hunter. In addition, pangolins possess a coronavirus that is almost similar to SARS-CoV-2 in one important region of its genome and may have been acquired from bats years ago. However, there is currently no proof that pangolins were present at the Wuhan market or even that the traders there engaged in pangolin trafficking. Mark Denison, director of pediatric infectious diseases at the Institute for Infection, Immunology, and

Inflammation at Vanderbilt University Medical Center, told me, "Somehow, we've created circumstances in our world that allow these viruses, which would otherwise not be known to cause any problems, to get into human populations." This particular virus just so happened to say, "I really like it here."

While the number of viable particles starts to decline within minutes, certain virus particles may survive for up to four hours on copper, twenty-four hours on cardboard, and seventy-two hours on plastic and stainless steel, according to researchers at Rocky Mountain Laboratories.

The new coronavirus is a deadly phantom. Much about this strain is still unknown since it has never been seen before. However, in just a few weeks, researchers have learned a remarkable amount—especially about how to treat or eradicate it through social distancing measures, antiviral medications, and, eventually, a vaccine—thanks to genetic detective work, atomic-level imaging, computer modeling, and earlier research on other coronavirus types, such as SARS and MERS (Middle East Respiratory Syndrome). Since January, about 800 publications dealing with the virus have been published on BIORxiv, a preprint platform for unreviewed research. Public databases now include over a thousand coronavirus genome sequences from various instances worldwide. Professor Kristian Andersen of Scripps Research's Department of Immunology and Microbiology told me, "It's crazy. Almost the whole scientific community is focused on this virus presently. We are discussing a scenario akin to a war.

 We are surrounded by many viruses that are composed of either DNA or RNA. DNA viruses, which are much more prevalent worldwide, may produce endemic, latent, and chronic systemic disorders. Examples of these include the papilloma viruses that cause cancer, the herpes viruses that cause chicken pox, and hepatitis B. According to Denison, "DNA viruses are the ones that live with us and stay with us." Retroviruses, such as H.I.V., contain RNA in their genomes but act like DNA viruses in their host, hence they are "lifelong." In contrast, RNA viruses are more quickly mutated and have simpler structures. Epstein told me that viruses can retain advantageous traits and mutate quickly. "A virus that is more promiscuous, more generalist, and that can inhabit and propagate in lots of other hosts ultimately has a better chance of surviving." Measles, Ebola, Zika, and a variety of respiratory infections, including influenza and coronaviruses, are among the viruses that frequently cause epidemics. "They're the ones that surprise us the most and do the most damage," said Paul Turner, a Yale University ecology and evolutionary biology professor who studied under Rachel Carson.

In the 1950s, researchers used early electron microscopes to examine samples from hens with infectious bronchitis and made the discovery of the coronavirus family. One of the three types of proteins that envelop the coronavirus's genetic code, or RNA, adorns the virus's surface with spikes that resemble mushrooms, earning it the name "crown." In the middle of the 1960s, researchers discovered two more coronaviruses that caused the common cold in humans after discovering further ones that afflicted pigs and cows. (Later, further screening found two more human coronaviruses that cause colds.) These four common cold viruses may have originated from animals in the past, but they are today exclusively human viruses that cause 15–30% of the seasonal colds in a given year. Similar to how bats are the natural reservoir for hundreds of other coronaviruses, we are their natural reservoir. However, they were mostly disregarded since they did not seem to cause serious illness. A meeting for nidovirales, the taxonomic group that includes coronaviruses, was almost canceled in 2003 because of low interest. Then SARS appeared, spreading from civets to bats to humans. The conference was completely sold out.

The new virus we are presently dealing with is closely similar to SARS. SARS primarily infects the lower respiratory system (the lungs), resulting in a far more deadly disease with a fatality rate of about 10%, whereas common-cold coronaviruses tend to infect only the upper respiratory tract (mainly the nose and throat), making them highly contagious. (MERS, which first appeared in Saudi Arabia in 2012 and spread from bats to camels to humans, also caused severe lower respiratory system disease and had a 37% fatality rate.) SARS-CoV-2 functions as a monstrous mutant hybrid of all the human coronaviruses that preceded it. It has the ability to spread throughout our airways. Stanley Perlman, a professor of microbiology and immunology who has spent more than thirty years researching coronaviruses, told me, "That is why it is so bad. It has the transmissibility of cold coronaviruses and the lower respiratory severity of SARS and MERS coronaviruses."

SARS-CoV-2's unique ability to attach and fuse with lung cells may be one factor contributing to its adaptability and, therefore, its success. Through a convoluted, multi-step process, all coronaviruses enter human cells using their spike proteins. First, if one visualizes the spike as a mushroom, the cap functions as a molecular key that fits into the locks of our cells. Researchers refer to these locks as receptors. The cap of SARS-CoV-2 attaches flawlessly to an ACE-2 receptor, which is present in the kidney cells and lungs, among other areas of the human body. Because their ACE-2 receptors are so open to the environment, coronaviruses target the respiratory system. Perlman informed me, "The virus simply jumps in, but it's difficult to reach the kidney."

Kizzmekia Corbett, the scientific lead of the coronavirus program at the National Institutes of Health Vaccine Research Center, told me that although the first SARS virus is also attached to the ACE-2 receptor, SARS-CoV-2 binds to it ten times more efficiently. "The binding is tighter, which could potentially mean that the beginning of the infection process is just more efficient." Additionally, SARS-CoV-2 appears to have a unique ability that SARS and MERS did not have: the ability to use enzymes from our human tissue, including furin, a common enzyme found in our bodies, to sever the spike protein's cap from its stem. Only then will the stem be able to join the membranes of the virus and the human cell, enabling the virus to spit its RNA into the cell. This enhanced capacity to attach to the ACE-2 receptor and use human enzymes to initiate fusion "could aid a lot in the transmissibility of this new virus and in seeding infections at a higher level," according to Lisa Gralinski, an assistant professor in the Department of Epidemiology at the University of North Carolina at Chapel Hill.

A coronavirus quickly multiplies after entering a human, where it hides in the upper respiratory tract and takes over the hardware of the cell. Since most RNA viruses lack a proofreading mechanism, their replication in a host is speedy and messy. Random and frequent mutations may result from this. However, Andersen informed me that "the great majority of those mutations just kill the virus immediately." However, coronaviruses do have the ability to check for faults during replication, unlike other RNA viruses. According to Denison, "they have an enzyme that actually corrects mistakes."

The presence of this enzyme, which turns coronaviruses into clever mutators, was first verified in research on live viruses by Denison's team at Vanderbilt. When there is no selection pressure to change, the viruses may stay stable in their host, but when they do, they can quickly develop. For instance, each time they jump into a new species, they may quickly change to adapt to the new environment, which includes a new immune system to fight and a new physiology. However, the virus adopts the mindset of "I'm happy, I'm good, no need to change" once it is readily propagating inside a species, according to Denison. Humans seem to be experiencing that right now; although SARS-CoV-2 strains vary somewhat throughout the world, none of them appear to have an impact on the virus's behavior. "This virus isn't changing very quickly. It's comparable to the finest Indianapolis 500 vehicle. There is nothing in its way, and it is in front. Therefore, there is no advantage to replacing the vehicle.

In order to release its viral genome and take control of the cell's machinery to replicate its RNA and produce new viral proteins, the coronavirus attaches itself to host cells and merges with their membrane. New virus particles made of proteins and RNA are released from the cell to infect more cells.

A virus multiplies in order to release large amounts of mucus, snot, phlegm, and even our breath from its host as quickly as possible. This allows the virus to continue spreading. As it happens, the coronavirus is an excellent shedder. Earlier this month, a German preprint study—one of the first outside of China to analyze data from patients with a COVID-19 diagnosis—found unmistakable proof that infected individuals shed the coronavirus at high rates prior to exhibiting symptoms. The virus effectively dons an invisibility cloak, maybe as a result of its enhanced capacity to attach and fuse to human cells. According to a new assessment by scientists, mildly symptomatic COVID-19 infections or unreported cases are 55% as infectious as severe ones. According to a different research, individuals who had more severe infections (that required hospitalization) had the virus in their respiratory tracts for up to 37 days.

A virus in parasitical purgatory, which is outside of a host, is inert—not quite living, but also not dead. Usually, hundreds or tens of thousands of coronavirus particles are required to infect an animal or a human, but a hundred million particles might fit on the tip of a pin and could survive for extended periods of time. According to researchers at the National Institute of Allergy and Infectious Diseases' Rocky Mountain Laboratories' Virus Ecology Unit in Montana, the virus can persist on copper for four hours, a piece of cardboard for twenty-four hours, and plastic or stainless steel for up to three days. Additionally, they discovered that the virus may float in the air for three hours and spread by the small respiratory droplets that an infected person coughs, sneezes, or exhales. (Other studies indicate that the virus may be able to survive as an aerosol, but only under very specific circumstances.) The majority of virus particles seem to lose their virulence quite rapidly. The first 10 minutes have the greatest infection window. Nevertheless, it seems sense that many of us have become germaphobes due to the possibility of illness.

Through the mouth, eyes, and nose, the coronavirus enters the body. From there, it travels to the lungs, where its particles multiply. The main way that HPV spreads to other people is by sneezing and coughing.

A virus just needs an unending supply of hosts. The ultimate aim of evolution is contagion. According to current investigations, scientists believe that COVID-19 is less contagious than the most contagious viruses, such as measles, which can spread to around twelve individuals from a single infected person, and somewhat more contagious than the typical flu. People who are almost completely asymptomatic yet distribute the coronavirus to a large number of others are probably super-spreaders. However, it is currently hard to pinpoint a precise infection rate. Denison said, "We often look to these absolute figures to tell us how concerned we should be." It's like floods, you see. Do you know whether it reaches my chin or my knees? It makes no difference. I have to take some action to attempt to prevent my automobile from colliding with the water.

We've already driven into the water in a lot of locations. Hospitals are running out of ventilators, beds, and supplies as hundreds of patients pass away every day. According to what scientists now know, a haywire immune response to the virus may be more responsible for the sickness in these severe COVID-19 patients than anything else. According to Perlman, the virus "basically beats the immune system to the punch and starts replicating too rapidly" since it can infiltrate our lower respiratory system while still donning its invisibility cloak. Since the immune system lacks particular antibodies to combat these unfamiliar new invaders, it may fly into overdrive and launch an offensive when it eventually detects their existence. Denison described it to me as "like dumping gas on the fire." The lung tissue fills with fluid and expands. Both breathing and oxygen exchange are inhibited. "The body kind of goes into shock because the host immune response is triggered to such an extreme level and then keeps building on itself," Gralinski said. The immune system is targeting areas of the body that shouldn't be attacked, which is similar to an autoimmune illness.

As with the 2003 SARS epidemic, this kind of reaction may be the reason why older people are generally more susceptible to COVID-19. When studying SARS in mice models, Denison told me that he had seen a phenomenon known as "immune senescence," in which older mice no longer had the capacity to respond in a balanced way to a new virus; their immune systems' overreaction then caused even more severe disease. There were almost no deaths among children under the age of thirteen during that outbreak, and when children did get sick, the disease was, on average, milder than what affected adults. According to Denison, this also happened in some of the worst cases during the first SARS epidemic, which explains why antiviral medications could be far more beneficial in the beginning of disease, before the immune system has had a chance to do its damage.

Denison's group and colleagues at the University of North Carolina have spent the last ten years investigating antiviral therapies in an effort to discover a cure that would not only combat SARS and MERS but also a new coronavirus that they predicted would eventually surface. Together, they conducted a large portion of the early research on Remdesivir, a medication presently being developed by Gilead and used in infected patient trials, as well as NHC, another antiviral medicinal molecule. In animal models, both medications were able to prevent the coronavirus from effectively reproducing in the body by avoiding, blocking, or circumventing its proofreading mechanism. "They performed exceptionally well against every coronavirus we tested," Denison informed me.

Since coronaviruses are enormous—among the biggest RNA viruses in the world—and need a method to preserve the structure of their lengthy genomes, it seems plausible that they include that proofreading enzyme. According to Andersen, the advantage of having such a large genome from our point of view "is that the more genes and protein products a virus has, the more opportunities we have to design specific treatments against them." For example, the virus's special capacity to use the human enzyme furin holds promise for antiviral medications that function as furin inhibitors.

Despite being relatively new to human hosts, COVID-19 will continue to cause a great deal of illness and fatalities. However, Epstein said, "Viruses tend to cause less severe disease over time as they evolve with their natural habitats." And that is beneficial for both the virus and the host. While the surviving hosts may develop some protection, the most virulent strains may burn out, which would result in many more terrible deaths. The stability of the virus—how much it is flourishing among us at the moment and just slightly changing—is more immediate and urgent, and it speaks well for the effectiveness of antiviral medications and, ultimately, a vaccine. Hospitals and medical personnel should experience some respite if the increasing number of mitigating measures—this historic national and worldwide shutdown—are maintained for a sufficient amount of time. "Our teacher is the virus," Denison informed me. It evolved throughout thousands of years to reach its current state. Right now, we're simply trying to catch up.

Facts About Remdesivir

Gilead Sciences, the massive antiviral producer with its headquarters located in Foster City, California, had a successful month in October. On October 8, the business signed a contract that might be worth over $1 billion to supply the European Union with its medication, remdesivir, which is used to treat COVID-19. On October 22, two weeks later, the U.S. Remdesivir became the first medication to be licensed by the Food and Drug Administration (FDA) for use against the pandemic coronavirus SARS-CoV-2 in the United States. Gilead's medication may now enter two significant markets with rising COVID-19 cases thanks to judgments made by the US and the EU.

However, both choices perplexed experts who have been carefully following Remdesivir's clinical studies over the last six months and who have numerous doubts about the drug's value. Remdesivir, at best, slightly shortened the recovery period from COVID-19 in hospitalized patients with severe disease, according to a large, well planned trial. A few smaller trials indicated that therapy had no effect at all on the condition. The fourth and largest controlled study then delivered what some considered a coup de grâce on October 15, amid this month's unfavorable news for Gilead: the World Health Organization's (WHO) Solidarity trial revealed that remdesivir does not lower mortality or the recovery time for COVID-19 patients.

Science has discovered that the corporation benefited greatly from the unique circumstances that led to both the FDA's decision and the EU agreement. A panel of independent specialists that the FDA has on hand to provide advice on complex antiviral medication matters has never been contacted. In order to review all available data on experimental treatments and recommend drug approvals to the FDA, the Antimicrobial Drugs Advisory Committee (AMDAC), which consists of infectious disease clinicians, biostatisticians, pharmacists, and a consumer representative, has not met once during the pandemic.

Meanwhile, precisely one week prior to the poor Solidarity study findings, the European Union agreed on the Remdesivir cost. Although Gilead, which had given Remdesivir to the study, was notified of the data on September 23 and knew the trial was a failure, it was not aware of those findings.

"This is a very, very bad look for the FDA, and the dealings between Gilead and EU make it another layer of badness," says Eric Topol, a Scripps Research Translational Institute cardiologist who opposed the FDA's approval of Remdesivir.

David Hardy, an HIV/AIDS scientist at the University of California, Los Angeles and a member of AMDAC, emphasizes that the FDA is not required to hold external panels for its determinations. However, the government often does so for complex medicine applications, and

Hardy is "amazed" that the panel wasn't consulted in this instance. "This sets the standard for the first COVID-19 antiviral," according to him. "When it comes to the point of giving pharmaceutical companies exclusive marketing rights in this area, that really is something that's very, very important. And there does need to be more than just governmental input."

Science asked FDA to explain why it chose not to form the committee, but FDA merely replied that it is "at the discretion" of division heads. However, the FDA's handling of possible COVID-19 vaccinations contrasts sharply with its inactivity. The FDA held an advisory group last week to talk about the potential for such a vaccination to pass regulatory muster.

According to Gilead, WHO sent the business a manuscript about the research results in "late September" regarding the EU accord. However, a representative for the European Commission, the EU executive branch, said that these findings were not disclosed during the talks. Due in part to the fact that the research was conducted in wildly disparate nations with varying levels of healthcare, the corporation has vigorously questioned the veracity of the Solidarity data. Gilead even went so far as to note in a statement dated October 15 that "it is unclear if any conclusive findings can be drawn from the study results."

The Solidarity study's scientists, notably Marie-Paule Kieny, a former WHO executive and head of research at the French medical research organization INSERM, are incensed by that critique. "It's appalling to see how Gilead tries to badmouth the Solidarity trial," adds Kieny. "Pretending the trial has no value because it is in low-income countries is just prejudice."

e
Remdesivir demonstrated strong inhibitory effects on the related coronavirus that causes Middle East respiratory syndrome in both test tube and mouse studies, according to a study

published in Nature Communications on January 10, two days after SARS-CoV-2 was identified as the cause of COVID-19. Two weeks later, medical professionals used the medication to treat the first verified instance of COVID-19 in the US, and they said the 35-year-old man quickly recovered.

On April 29, the National Institutes of Health (NIH) released an interim analysis from a large-scale, placebo-controlled clinical study that raised hopes but also highlighted remdesivir's potential. The medication shortened the median recovery period for hospitalized, critically sick COVID-19 patients from 15 days to 11 days. Remdesivir, which must be repeatedly administered intravenously, also seemed to reduce the risk of mortality, although the difference may have been due to chance. The NIH said in a news release that treated patients "had a 31% faster time to recovery than those who received placebo." (The study's final, peer-reviewed report, which was published on October 8 in The New England Journal of

Medicine, shortened the recovery period for the 531 patients who received treatment to 10 days.)

Remdesivir did not show any statistically significant advantage in a second, smaller, placebo-controlled trial of the drug on hospitalized COVID-19 patients in China, which was also published online by The Lancet on April 29. Surprisingly, the antiviral drug had no effect on coronavirus levels.

Remdesivir received an emergency use authorization (EUA), a provisional status that is far from full approval, from the FDA for treatment in patients with severe COVID-19 two days after the findings from China and the US were released. The second research was not acknowledged by the FDA, but the NIH trial data was. During a news conference in the Oval Office, President Donald Trump commended the EUA alongside Gilead CEO Daniel O'Day.

Gilead's attempts to disparage the Solidarity trial are disgusting. It is only prejudice to act as

if the trial is worthless because it takes place in a low-income country.
   Kieny, Marie-Paule, INSERM

   In a study funded by Gilead and published online in JAMA on August 21, hospitalized COVID-19 patients with mild pneumonia who were given remdesivir for five or ten days were compared to those who received conventional treatment. Strangely, the 10-day group did not improve as soon as the 5-day remdesivir group did. (There was no difference between the two treatment regimens in a previous published trial that was funded by Gilead.)

   Remdesivir's EUA was extended by the FDA the following week to include all hospitalized COVID-19 patients. As a result, Topol, the editor-in-chief of the well-known medical website Medscape, sent a damning open letter to FDA Commissioner Stephen Hahn. Under the heading "Tell the Truth or Resign," Topol grouped the ruling with highly criticized EUAs previously awarded for antibody-rich "convalescent" plasma drawn from the blood of recovered COVID-19 patients and the malaria medication hydroxychloroquine, which the agency subsequently revoked. "These repeated breaches demonstrate your willingness to ignore the lack of scientific evidence, and to be complicit with the Trump Administration's politicization of America's healthcare institutions," Topol said.

Disputes about the evidence

Many experts anticipated that the WHO's Solidarity study, which was carried out in 405 hospitals across 30 countries, would better determine the value of Remdesivir since it was about three times as big as the other three studies combined. Instead of using a placebo, Solidarity compared Remdesivir and three other repurposed medications against the standard of therapy and to each other. On October 10, the Solidarity trial scientists presented the research data to FDA officials. Five days later, they published a preprint on medRxiv. None of the medications reduced mortality among hospitalized COVID-19 patients, which was the primary goal of Solidarity. Remdesivir had no effect on "the duration of hospitalization" or whether COVID-19 patients needed ventilators, which are only used when a patient's condition worsened, according to the study.

 The Solidarity data's publication has sparked a new discussion over the relative merits of each Remdesivir study and whether the FDA ought to have discussed the issue publicly rather than behind closed doors. The government ignored the Solidarity data and the results of the second placebo-controlled trial in China, and only included data from three studies in its analysis that suggested remdesivir's approval: the NIH study and two Gilead-sponsored trials.

 The Solidarity crew was furious about it. "The mantra I've always heard as a joke about the FDA is that they say 'In God we trust, everyone else has to provide data,'" says Kieny. "So look at all the data."

The Solidarity statistics shouldn't be significant from Gilead's perspective. "We are concerned that the data from this open-label global trial have not undergone the rigorous review required to allow for constructive scientific discussion, particularly given the limitations of the trial design," the business said in a statement.

The idea that the sooner you utilize it, the better, is a nice one, unless you consider the consequences: You will have to treat a lot of people and you won't save many lives. It will cost you a lot and is incredibly inconvenient.
Oxford University's Martin Landray

Solidarity "does not negate other study results—particularly from a trial designed with the strictest of scientific standards, as is the case with" NIH's study, according to an open letter written by Gilead Chief Medical Officer Merdad Parsey and published on the day the FDA approved Remdesivir. Gilead has also questioned whether Solidarity's data is readily available, telling Science that it has asked WHO for "the underlying data sets or statistical analysis plan" for the experiment but has not yet received it.

WHO responds that Gilead will get the whole data set when the research is finished and was aware of the statistical analysis approach before to enrolling in the trial. WHO experts claim that because the FDA has a history of reviewing all available data, including unpublished results, it makes no difference that the data have not yet undergone peer review. WHO top scientist Soumya Swaminathan points out that 50% of the 2750 patients who took remdesivir in the study were from Canada and Europe, two regions known for providing high-quality healthcare, in response to Gilead's claim that the differences in health systems constitute a complicating issue in Solidarity's results. She also emphasizes that subpar treatment is not always present in the other participating nations.

The primary difference between Solidarity and the NIH research, according to Clifford Lane of the National Institute of Allergy and Infectious Diseases, is "the degree of granularity" of the analysis of subgroups that would have benefitted. According to Lane, "I think the Solidarity data are fine," "It's a very large study and it has a very robust endpoint."

Remdesivir "definitely doesn't work in the sickest patients where the biggest gains would be," according to Martin Landray of the University of Oxford, who is co-leading the largest trial of several COVID-19 medications in the world. However, he suggests that it could benefit patients at an earlier stage of the illness. To make matters more complicated, the majority of SARS-CoV-2 infections resolve on their own. "The argument that the earlier you use it the better is great until you realize what the implications of that are: You won't save many lives, and you'll have to treat a lot of patients," Landray explains. "It's very inconvenient, and it'll cost you a fortune."

Concerns have also been raised about Remdesivir's potential for damage. The World Health Organization regularly reviews potential adverse medication events associated with COVID-19 therapy. Remdesivir individuals reported a disproportionately high incidence of liver and renal issues in late August as compared to those getting other COVID-19 medications. This month, the European Medicines Agency (EMA) also revealed that its safety committee has begun an evaluation to evaluate allegations of acute kidney damage in some remdesivir-using patients.

Numerous experts point out that the FDA's statement about Remdesivir's clearance completely omits another important piece of information: proof that the medication lowers the viral load, or the quantity of SARS-CoV-2 in the body. "Every time you study an antiviral, you show an effect on the virus and you publish it," says Andrew Hill, a clinical pharmacologist at the University of Liverpool. "I've been working in antivirals for 30 years." "Surely

Gilead has done that. Where are the data? It is very, very strange."

The WHO experiment cannot demonstrate that remdesivir has no benefit for COVID-19, according to Richard Peto, an epidemiologist and statistician from Oxford who assisted in the design of Solidarity and conducted the data analysis. "Trials produce confidence intervals, not just point estimates and this is actually the difficulty in trying to discuss this," adds Peto. "Gilead and the FDA have sort of maneuvered us into a position where we're being asked to try and prove remdesivir does nothing rather than asking the usual way round, which is, 'Can the manufacturers prove it does something?'"

These intricacies, in the opinion of many scientists, highlight the need for the FDA to engage in a robust discussion with its panel of independent experts, ADAC. This may have "elevated the discussion," according to Brigham and Women's Hospital infectious disease expert Lindsey Baden, chair of the ADAC.

"Hydroxychloroquine, convalescent plasma, remdesivir—these are complicated decisions given the imperfect nature of the data upon which the decisions are being made, and the urgency of the clinical use gives all the more reasons to have an open discussion," says Baden, whose group met for the last time in October 2019.

"This was not a straightforward approval and this is not an ordinary time," the FDA's former acting head scientist Luciana Borio, who is now employed by a non-profit venture capital business, adds. "It would have been helpful to have a public discussion on the matter."

Jesse Goodman, a former FDA top scientist at Georgetown University, said that although setting up advisory committee meetings is difficult, the FDA clearly recently set one up for COVID-19 vaccines. "Although it's a pandemic and everybody is super busy, it's something … you can do virtually," he claims. "It would have been an opportunity to make clear publicly the rationale and their risk-benefit assessment."

The European Commission is unaware of

Remdesivir received "conditional approval" in July from Europe's FDA equivalent, the European Medicines Agency (EMA), which is comparable to an EUA, although it has not yet granted its complete clearance. Nevertheless, the European Union and Gilead have signed a "joint procurement agreement" that promises 500,000 treatment sessions for $1.2 billion over the next six months. According to a Commission spokeswoman, Science was not notified of the drug's failure in the Solidarity trial until the day after the signing of the new contract on October 8.

"The Commission became aware of the results of the Solidarity trial on 9 October from the reporting of [EMA] at the COVID task force meeting on the same day," according to a spokeswoman. "There was no discussion with WHO about the ongoing study prior to signing the contract with Gilead."

Gilead acknowledged receiving a draft manuscript from WHO in late September, but said it was "heavily redacted." According to WHO, the only information blacked out was results relating to the other drugs used in the trial because of confidentiality agreements with their manufacturers. This was in response to Science's question about why Gilead had not disclosed the Solidarity data during its negotiations with the Commission.

This permission was not simple, and this is not a typical moment. A public debate on the issue would have been beneficial.

Former FDA acting chief scientist Luciana Borio

A spokesman for the Commission told Science that although the deal with Gilead binds EU nations to paying around $2400 for a course of Remdesivir, it does not require any nation to buy the medication. According to Yannis Natsis of the European Public Health Alliance, a nonprofit organization, "the EU needs to publish the deal with Gilead." Gilead maintains it has no intention of changing its agreed pricing in response to the Solidarity statistics, but "it should at least renegotiate the volume of the doses and the price per treatment."

Kieny claims that the EU's investment on Remdesivir, which is predicated on the theory that it would benefit a tiny percentage of patients, is a "enormous" waste. "You can always say, 'OK, now, if I disaggregate the population and if I take only those who have a blue eye and a wooden leg, maybe this is very effective,'" she continues.

Remdesivir proponents do, in fact, cite Solidarity patient subgroup studies that indicate a mortality advantage for those who were not on ventilators but got supplementary oxygen.

However, acknowledging that would also include acknowledging that remdesivir caused damage to ventilator users, according to Hill. "You can't do a subgroup analysis and only believe half the story."

According to Jason Pogue, a researcher at the University of Michigan, Ann Arbor, and president of the Society of Infectious Diseases Pharmacists, the conclusion drawn from the studies so far is that there is just insufficient proof that remdesivir is effective. Pogue thinks the FDA erred and that EMA shouldn't fully approve the medication until further information is available. "There are more questions than answers about the efficacy of remdesivir in hospitalized patients," according to him.

The COVID Heart

An examination of data from around 154 000 US veterans infected with SARS-CoV-2 offers a sobering first response to the query: What are the long-term cardiovascular consequences of COVID-19? In the year following recovery from the acute phase of the illness, patients were more likely to experience a variety of cardiovascular issues, such as irregular heartbeats, inflammation of the heart muscle, blood clots, strokes, myocardial infarction, and heart failure, according to a study published in Nature Medicine by researchers at the Veterans Affairs (VA) St. Louis Health Care System. Furthermore, the increased risks were noticeable even for those without acute COVID-19 hospitalization.

The History

In an email to JAMA, study senior author Ziyad Al-Aly, MD, said that the research team decided to find and fill significant information gaps about COVID-19 at the start of the epidemic. Al-Aly, a clinical epidemiologist at Washington University in St. Louis and head of research and development at the VA St. Louis Health Care System, said, "At that time, none of us knew anything about long COVID." "Over a period of weeks, we began to hear about patients who were not fully recovering and had lingering issues, including heart problems." The team was motivated to investigate long COVID, sometimes referred to as post-COVID disorders, by these patients, who identify as long carriers.

Researchers showed that individuals with prolonged COVID may have complications in several organ systems, including cardiovascular diseases, in a work that was published in Nature in April. They want to better understand the long-term cardiovascular effects of COVID-19 with the present investigation.

The layout

A thorough, predetermined set of cardiovascular outcomes among US Veterans Health Administration (VHA) system patients who survived the first 30 days of COVID-19 were the focus of the recent research published in Nature Medicine. Using data from three sizable cohorts' electronic medical records, the researchers calculated the risks and extra burden of cardiovascular events per 1000 people 12 months following COVID-19:

Between March 1, 2020, and January 15, 2021, 153,760 patients who received VHA services in 2019 and got a positive SARS-CoV-2 test result

The modern control group consists of 5637 647 patients who used VHA services in 2019 and showed no signs of SARS-CoV-2 infection.

The historical control group consisted of 5 859 411 prepandemic individuals who used VHA services in 2017.

Older White male patients made up the majority of the cohorts. 89% of the COVID-19 cohort, which had an average age of 61, were men, and almost 71% were white. However, due to the study's size, it also included almost 17,000 female patients, about 37,000 Black patients, and nearly 8,000 COVID-19 patients who were Latino, Asian, American Indian, Native Hawaiian, and of other races.

What We've Discovered

Numerous cardiovascular conditions, including as cerebrovascular disorders, dysrhythmias, ischemic and non-ischemic heart disease, pericarditis, myocarditis, heart failure, and thromboembolic disease, were more likely to occur in patients with COVID-19.

At the 12-month point, for every 1000 individuals, COVID-19 was linked to an additional of the following:

45.29 instances of any cardiovascular event that was predetermined

Major adverse cardiovascular events (MACEs), such as myocardial infarction, stroke, and all-cause death, occurred in 23.48 cases.

10.74 cases of atrial fibrillation were among the 19.86 dysrhythmia events.

There were 12.72 cases of various cardiovascular conditions, including 3.56 cases of nonischemic cardiomyopathy and 11.61 cases of heart failure.
9.88 cases of thromboembolic diseases, including 4.18 cases of deep vein thrombosis and 5.47 cases of pulmonary embolism

7.28 cases of ischemic heart disease, including 2.91 myocardial infarction cases, 2.5 angina episodes, and 5.35 cases of acute coronary disease

4.03 stroke events and 5.48 cases of cerebrovascular illnesses

1.23 cases of pericardial or cardiac inflammatory illness, including 0.98 cases of pericarditis and 0.31 cases of myocarditis

Higher risks were associated with patients who had more severe illness, as indicated by whether they were admitted to the critical care unit, hospitalized, or recovered at home. However, even among those who were not hospitalized with COVID-19, the dangers were apparent. Regardless of age, race, sex, obesity, smoking, hypertension, diabetes, chronic renal disease, hyperlipidemia, and prior cardiovascular disease, other subgroup analyses revealed elevated risks.

When comparing the results of patients with COVID-19 to those of the prepandemic control group, the study's overall conclusions were in agreement.

A Remark on Heart Disease

The authors performed studies to exclude the impact of immunization since some COVID-19 vaccinations may be linked to uncommon instances of myocarditis and pericarditis. Regardless of immunization status, the elevated risk of myocarditis and pericarditis persisted among unvaccinated individuals.

The Unexpected

The extent of cardiovascular disease involvement was "eye opening," according to Al-Aly's email, while the elevated chances were particularly noticeable for heart failure and atrial fibrillation. The higher risks seen for those who were not hospitalized for COVID-19 during the acute phase—the group that comprises the majority of those infected with SARS-CoV-2—also caught the researchers off guard. The study did not, however, examine symptomatic vs asymptomatic infections, which may be a topic for future investigation.

According to Al-Aly, the subgroup analyses also produced unexpected findings. "But the data showed that COVID-19 may be an equal opportunity offender," he said, contradicting his initial assumption that the health problems would be obvious among those at high risk of cardiovascular disease. "Young people and old people, Black people and white people, men and women, smokers and nonsmokers, people with diabetes and those without, etc., were all at risk." No grouping was spared, in fact.

Al-Aly pointed out that preclinical cardiovascular illness and cardiovascular hazards, such obesity and chronic renal disease, may have contributed to certain people's poorer cardiovascular outcomes after COVID-19 and raised their likelihood of contracting

SARS-CoV-2 infection in the first place. The elevated risk in every research subgroup, however, "probably indicates that infection with SARS-CoV-2 is also causing de novo cardiovascular disease," he concluded.

The Clinical Conclusion

A history of COVID-19 should be taken into account by doctors as a risk factor for cardiovascular disease. Al-Aly noted, "We believe it is critical to closely monitor individuals with COVID-19 and detect early signs or symptoms of heart disease." He underlined that reducing the likelihood of more serious downstream health effects would need early detection, diagnosis, and treatment.

How to Identify the COVID Heart

According to Al-Aly, the research shows that cardiovascular disease is one aspect of the complex illness known as protracted COVID.

He underlined that long-term COVID is more than just exhaustion or mental fog; it's the collection of symptoms and organ dysfunction brought on by COVID-19 that continue or reappear throughout the postacute stage of the illness.

Al-Aly described the effort as a "long COVID moonshot," stating that a coordinated worldwide response plan is urgently required to meet the difficulties of addressing the long-term health impacts of COVID-19 as the epidemic approaches its third year.
In order to better understand the health trajectories and long-term consequences of individuals with cardiovascular COVID, he said, "I believe there are a lot of knowledge gaps that need to be investigated in future research." Future study is crucial in determining the most effective ways to recognize, diagnose, and treat these people.

Arizona University:

The University of Arizona (UA) became a complicated case study in both innovation and controversy during the COVID-19 epidemic. UA stood out in the early stages of the epidemic because to its innovative scientific approach. By developing a technique for identifying viral RNA in sewage, wastewater testing on campus enabled it to spot outbreaks in student residence halls before any symptoms showed up. More widespread illnesses among staff and kids were probably avoided by this preventative action. Additionally, UA researchers put a lot of effort into advancing public health knowledge by evaluating COVID-19 studies to get a better understanding of the virus and to rectify false information that was being spread in public and scientific discourse. These steps created a powerful impression of a research-based organization using evidence-based tactics to combat the epidemic.

However, there were serious administrative and budgetary challenges hidden beneath the well-publicized successes. The institution imposed drastic financial cutbacks, including teaching and staff furloughs and salary reductions, when COVID-19 struck. Critics noted that UA made the extremely contentious choice to acquire Ashford University, a failed for-profit online institution, when these austerity measures were being implemented. Despite internal concerns regarding Ashford's low academic reputation, declining enrollment, and legal difficulties connected to fraudulent methods, this deal was accomplished and Ashford was rebranded as the University of Arizona Global Campus. The decision, which put UA's finances under even more pressure during the epidemic, was seen by many faculty members and outsiders as a financial risk motivated more by desperation than strategic planning.

During this period, there was also a decline in the administration-student interaction at the institution, particularly among graduate students. Graduate students said that policies were being handed down without enough consultation or consideration of their safety and financial well-being, and they sought more openness and influence into pandemic decision-making. Public tensions erupted as a result of demonstrations and official complaints against the administration's COVID-related practices from some graduate organizations.

The problem was exacerbated by UA's approach to communicating about breakouts on campus. The management of the university sometimes seemed to blame students for the increases in infection, blaming them for gatherings and disobedience, as COVID-19 cases increased on campus, especially in the autumn of 2020. However, detractors—including The Daily Wildcat, UA's student newspaper—pointed out that the institution was not always following safety procedures and often sent conflicting signals about what conduct was appropriate, which added to the confusion and mayhem.

Students and employees felt that the administration's PR campaigns were more about preserving the university's reputation and budget than they were about really putting health and safety first.

In terms of science, a few of UA's specialists also contributed to the larger COVID-19 discussion on the virus's genesis. According to them, the "lab leak" notion that COVID-19 was created or unintentionally leaked from a laboratory was not supported by any reliable scientific data. In addition to stressing the need of concentrating on scientific data, UA experts cautioned that politicizing the virus's origins would undermine public confidence in science, which was already severely weakened during the epidemic.

When combined, the COVID-19 period at the University of Arizona told the tale of two worlds coexisting. On the one hand, it made a significant contribution to scientific study and innovation in the worldwide pandemic response.

However, serious weaknesses were exposed by contentious administrative choices, internal financial mismanagement, and a breakdown of confidence among the university community. While UA's public image during COVID-19 focused on leadership and scientific advancement, the "hidden truth" is that, behind the scenes, the university faced financial instability, dubious strategic choices, and strained relationships with its own students and staff—all of which were made worse by the pandemic's pressures.

The University of Arizona positioned itself as a pioneer in pandemic leadership and scientific innovation when COVID-19 struck. But beyond that well-preserved exterior, the reality was much more sloppy and awkward. Although UA received recognition for its innovative strategies, such as wastewater testing to identify COVID-19 outbreaks early, this achievement concealed severe internal problems, financial hardship, and a growing gulf between the academic community and the administration.

Prior to the epidemic, UA was already having financial difficulties. COVID-19 made matters worse, but UA leadership acted rashly rather than carefully tightening procedures. The most obvious was the purchase of Ashford University, an online institution beset by controversy and in decline. UA persisted in renaming Ashford the University of Arizona Global Campus even though it was aware that the institution was being investigated for dishonest business practices, had poor graduation rates, and was experiencing declining enrollment. This agreement was often seen as a lifeline for Ashford's corporate owners rather than for the reputation or students of UA. It indicated that the administration valued hazardous growth above addressing fundamental issues and immediately put an already tight university budget at danger.

Many employees and students felt abandoned within the institution. Graduate students at UA, who lead research and teach lectures, said they were treated like disposable labor. Despite being among those most at danger, they were mostly excluded from pandemic decision-making. Anger and resentment were stoked when their requests for better working conditions and financial safeguards were either disregarded or postponed. In the meanwhile, as administrators made costly, high-stakes decisions with minimal scrutiny, faculty members experienced furloughs and salary cutbacks.

Instead of taking responsibility for its own uneven regulations, UA's administration opted to blame students for outbreaks when COVID-19 cases spiked on campus. The administration often used conflicting language, urging children to return to school while downplaying the actual hazards and then reprimanding them when illnesses eventually surfaced. At best, safety regulations were not always strictly enforced. To protect themselves from criticism, UA's senior authorities blamed students for the planning and execution errors rather than taking responsibility for them.

The university has participated in the national discussion over the origins of COVID-19. In line with a scientific narrative that placed an emphasis on zoonotic origins, UA specialists openly disregarded the lab leak idea. Even while their scientific justifications made sense, several detractors saw this as part of a larger pattern in which colleges, which depend significantly on government money and research collaborations, were fast to follow the politically safe path during a period of intense divisiveness and censorship around COVID-related issues.

In summary, the University of Arizona, like many big institutions, made a concerted effort to preserve a public image of control, innovation, and community caring during COVID-19. On the inside, however, it was plagued by financial mismanagement, administrative irresponsibility, betrayal of its most vulnerable employees, and a decline in internal trust. These issues weren't caused by the epidemic; rather, it brought them to light, emphasized them, and made the institution face its true priorities: surviving at all costs, even at the expense of long-term stability, equity, and openness.

Issue with Clotting:

The coagulation system is significantly disrupted by COVID-19 for a number of reasons:

Direct viral impacts cause inflammation and damage to endothelial cells, which line blood arteries and increase their propensity to clot.

Clotting factors rise as a result of systemic inflammation brought on by the immune system's reaction, particularly the cytokine storm.

Blood clots in a variety of organs are caused by platelet activation and aggregation brought on by immune dysregulation.

2. Clot Types Observed in COVID-19
Blood clots that develop in veins, usually in the legs, are known as deep vein thrombosis (DVT).

Clots that migrate to the lungs, obstructing blood flow and resulting in respiratory discomfort, are known as pulmonary emboli (PE).

Stroke: The brain's blood supply may be cut off by blood clots.

Microclots: These microscopic clots may develop in the heart, brain, kidneys, lungs, and other organs, causing harm to those organs.

3. Important Data: COVID-19 Clotting Incidents
General Hospitalized Patients:
Blood clots may occur in as much as 30% of COVID-19 hospitalized patients.

ICU Patients: Up to 50% of critical cases result in thrombotic events, such as PE, DVT, and organ microclots.

D-dimer Levels: Patients with COVID-19 often have elevated D-dimer levels, which are indicative of clot formation and disintegration.

Severe consequences, including death, have been associated with elevated D-dimer levels.

ICU Clotting Risks from COVID-19:
49% of intensive care unit (ICU) patients had venous thromboembolism (VTE), which includes pulmonary embolism and deep vein thrombosis, according to a New York research.
(Reference: Klok and colleagues, 2020)

Thrombosis Risk: Compared to patients without thrombosis, ICU patients with thrombosis had a mortality risk that was more than twice as high.

Mortality and Clotting:
In cases with severe COVID-19, elevated D-dimer levels are a reliable indicator of death. According to a Chinese research, patients with higher D-dimer levels were four times more likely to die.
(Reference: Tang and colleagues, 2020)

Stroke Rate:
Two to six percent of hospitalized COVID-19 patients had a stroke. Compared to the typical 0.5% seen in the overall hospitalized population, this is much greater.

4. Clotting Mechanisms in COVID-19
Endothelial Impairment:
By directly infecting endothelial cells, COVID-19 damages the lining of blood vessels. Increased permeability and clot development in the blood arteries result from this. In organs like the lungs, where clotting may exacerbate respiratory discomfort, this is particularly true.

Storm of Cytokines and Inflammation:
Pro-inflammatory cytokines (such as IL-6, IL-1, and TNF-alpha) and pro-coagulant proteins (such as fibrinogen, factor VIII, and vWF) are elevated in the cytokine storm brought on by COVID-19. This increases the body's coagulation.

Activation of Platelets:
During COVID-19, platelets, which typically aid in blood clotting after injury, become hyperactive. Platelet aggregation is improperly induced in COVID-19, which may cause thrombi to develop in veins and arteries.

Hypercoagulability
Patients with COVID-19 are hypercoagulable, which increases the risk of blood clotting because to:

increased levels of the clotting protein fibrinogen.

increased factor VIII, which hastens the production of clots.

diminished fibrinolysis, or the capacity to disintegrate clots.

5. Clotting Problems After COVID-19 (Long COVID)

Even months after infection, some COVID-19 individuals who recover still have clotting issues:

Long COVID: Research indicates that up to 30% of people with Long COVID may get microclots, which might exacerbate chronic symptoms including exhaustion, dyspnea, and mental haze.

Long-term effects on the coagulation system were shown by a research that found that 30 to 50% of patients had chronic clotting problems even after they recovered.

6. Vaccine-Induced Immune Thrombotic Thrombocytopenia, or VITT, is clotting in COVID-19 vaccines.

VITT: An immune response that activates platelets was associated with very uncommon blood clotting events that occurred after vaccinations such as those from AstraZeneca and Johnson & Johnson.

For AstraZeneca, the VITT rate was 1 in 1 million, whereas for Johnson & Johnson, it was 1 in 500,000.

Since this clotting condition is caused by autoimmune responses rather than viral infections, it differs from COVID-19-associated clotting.

7. Important Research on Clotting and COVID-19

According to Klok et al. (2020) in New York, blood clots formed in 30–50% of intensive care unit patients, and they were highly associated with unfavorable outcomes, including mortality.

According to Tang et al. (2020) from China, individuals with COVID-19 who have elevated D-dimer levels have a worse prognosis and a greater death rate.

According to Zuo et al. (2021), microclots continue to form even in individuals who have recovered from long-term COVID.

8. Treatments & Preventions for COVID-19 Clotting

Heparin and other anticoagulants are often administered to hospitalized patients in order to avoid the development of clots.

Blood thinner dosages are modified according to risk variables, such as infection severity and D-dimer levels.

Antiplatelet therapy: Aspirin and other medications are sometimes used, especially in individuals who have a high risk of clotting.

ongoing investigation on new anticoagulants and antiplatelet medicines designed especially to prevent clotting caused by COVID-19.

Key Points Synopsis:
A hypercoagulable condition brought on by COVID-19 increases the risk of clotting events such DVT, PE, and stroke.

Although milder instances may also be affected, clotting is more likely in severe and intensive care unit patients.

A significant indicator of increased clotting and a worse prognosis is elevated D-dimer levels.

Some post-COVID patients continue to have long-term clotting problems (Long COVID).

Although there is a rare risk of clotting (VITT) with vaccines, the advantages exceed the dangers.

Here's a snapshot of how serious clotting problems were in COVID-19 patients (based on studies from 2020–2022):

1. Deep Vein Thrombosis (DVT) and Pulmonary Embolism (PE)

In hospitalized COVID-19 patients, ~20–30% developed blood clots.

In ICU (critical care) patients, the rate was even higher — up to 50%.

Many clots formed despite patients being given blood thinners.

2. Microclots in Organs

Autopsies showed widespread microthrombi (tiny clots) in the lungs, heart, kidneys, and brain.

This partly explained why some patients had severe respiratory failure even when their lungs weren't "filled" with fluid like in typical pneumonia.

3. Stroke and Heart Attack

COVID-19 increased the risk of ischemic stroke (blockages in brain blood vessels), even in young people without traditional risk factors.

Some patients had heart attacks caused by clotting in the coronary arteries.

4. D-dimer Levels

D-dimer is a blood test that measures clot breakdown products.

In COVID-19 patients, high D-dimer levels strongly predicted poor outcomes.

If your D-dimer was elevated, your risk of death was much higher.

5. Vaccine-induced clotting (VITT)

Rare (like 1 case per 100,000–1,000,000 vaccinations), but serious.

More common with AstraZeneca and Johnson & Johnson vaccines.

Different mechanism than COVID-19 itself — an autoimmune attack on platelets.

In visual numbers (simplified): Population	% with clotting issues
Hospitalized COVID patients	20–30%
ICU COVID patients	30–50%

Non-hospitalized (mild COVID)	<5%

COVID-19 was a vascular illness in addition to a lung infection.

Through thromboinflammation (inflammation + clotting), it damaged blood vessels, induced excessive clotting, and resulted in harm to several organs.

Could Snakes Be The Original Source?

The recently identified coronavirus that has caused a catastrophic infectious respiratory disease epidemic in China this winter may have originated in snakes, namely the Chinese cobra and the Chinese krait.

A very poisonous elapid snake, the many-banded krait (Bungarus multicinctus) is distributed over most of central and southern China as well as Southeast Asia. It is sometimes referred to as the Chinese krait or the Taiwanese krait. CC BY-SA Briston/Wikimedia

The disease has been spreading quickly since it was first discovered in Wuhan, a large city in central China, in late December 2019. People in China and other nations, including the US, have since contracted the disease from ill Wuhan tourists.

Chinese researchers have identified the virus's genetic code and taken pictures of it under microscopes using samples of the virus that were isolated from patients. A novel coronavirus is the disease causing this pandemic. The well-known Middle East respiratory syndrome coronavirus (MERS-CoV) and severe acute respiratory syndrome coronavirus (SARS-CoV), which have killed hundreds of people over the last 17 years, belong to the same virus family. The novel coronavirus has been dubbed 2019-nCoV by the World Health Organization (WHO).

As journal editors and virologists, we are keeping a careful eye on this epidemic since there are a lot of concerns that need to be addressed in order to stop this public health hazard from spreading.

The symptoms of this novel 2019-CoV are comparable to those of SARS-CoV and MERS-CoV. A significant inflammatory reaction is seen by those infected with these coronaviruses.

Transmission of zoonotic diseases

Both MERS and SARS are categorized as zoonotic viral illnesses, which means that the first sick individuals got the viruses directly from animals. This was made feasible by the virus acquiring a number of genetic alterations while in the animal host, which enabled it to infect and proliferate inside humans.

These viruses may now spread from one person to another. According to field research, the bat is the primary source of both SARS-CoV and MERS-CoV, with camels and masked palm civets—two mammals endemic to Asia and Africa—acting as intermediary hosts between bats and humans.

According to reports, the majority of the initial patients admitted to the hospital during the 2019 coronavirus outbreak were employees or patrons of a nearby seafood wholesale market that also offered processed meats and live consumable animals, such as chickens, donkeys, sheep, pigs, camels, foxes, badgers, bamboo rats, hedgehogs, and reptiles. It is possible, however, that the coronavirus may have come from other animals sold in that market, given no one has ever reported discovering a coronavirus infecting aquatic species.

A recent article in the Journal of Medical Virology amply supports the theory that the 2019-nCoV jumped from an animal at the market. The genetic sequences of 2019-nCoV and every other coronavirus that is known were analyzed and compared by the researchers.

The new virus is most closely linked to two bat SARS-like coronavirus samples from China, according to an analysis of its genetic coding. This finding first raises the possibility that, like SARS and MERS, the bat may also be the genesis of 2019-nCoV. The investigators also discovered that the 2019-nCoV spike protein's DNA coding sequence suggests that the bat virus may have undergone a mutation before to infecting humans. This protein forms the "crown" of the viral particle, which identifies the receptor on a host cell.

However, a more thorough bioinformatics examination of the 2019-nCoV sequencing by the researchers indicates that this coronavirus may have originated in snakes.

From snakes to bats

The researchers analyzed the protein codes that the novel coronavirus preferred and contrasted them with those of coronaviruses that were identified in a variety of animal hosts, including humans, birds, snakes, marmots, hedgehogs, manis, and bats. They discovered, rather surprisingly, that the 2019-nCoV's protein codes are most like those seen in snakes.

In the wild, snakes often hunt bats. According to reports, snakes were offered for sale at Wuhan's local seafood market. This suggests that the 2019-nCoV may have spread from its host species, bats, to snakes and ultimately to people during the start of the coronavirus epidemic. It is yet unknown, however, how the virus may adjust to both warm-blooded and cold-blooded hosts.

Laboratory tests are required by the report's authors and other researchers to confirm the virus's origin. The first step would be to look for the 2019-nCoV sequence in snakes. However, the seafood market has been closed and sterilized since the outbreak, making it difficult to identify the animal that is the source of the new virus.

To verify the virus's origin, DNA samples from market animals as well as from wild snakes and bats must be collected. However, the published results will also provide valuable information for creating preventative and treatment plans.

Another reminder that humans should restrict their eating of wild animals in order to avoid zoonotic diseases is the 2019-nCoV epidemic.

Shereen's story: my lengthy COVID experience

In March 2020, Glasgow resident Shereen, 38, had her first severe episode of coronavirus, necessitating hospitalization.

"I remember thinking to myself that if I didn't have it, I would by the time I left." "When I saw the doctor, she wasn't wearing any PPE, and I was so worried for her and scared that I would be the one to infect her." "I was placed in a waiting room with many other people who had suspected COVID when I arrived at the hospital to be checked. That was a thought that played on my mind for weeks after that."

Shereen was sent home to her apartment in the city center, where she lives alone, after receiving a diagnosis just before regular testing.

"I was so sick, I felt like I was going to die. The symptoms of COVID are agony. I'm usually a very capable and self-sufficient person, but it felt like I had been to a war zone. In addition to the physical pain, I felt toxic. I was very aware of the risk of infecting others and made sure to isolate, even covering the letterbox with a plastic bag. After my initial illness, I hoped I would be on the mend, but I've suffered from relapses ever since. The first one occurred about three weeks later, and it felt like a scab was being torn off my lungs; they were burning. Nevertheless, it took me six months to return to the hospital I visited when I first contracted COVID in order to attend a respiratory clinic. I was so nervous about going back there that I had panic attacks.

Shereen's life is much quieter now than it was before, but she still feels the effects of long-term COVID, even though relapses are less frequent. She still has muscle and joint pain, for which she needs to take two nerve pain medications and see a physiotherapist, and she is unable to walk for more than 20 minutes or talk for extended periods of time without planning enough rest to prevent being totally exhausted.

Shereen was a singer before she became sick with COVID, and she was also prepared to start a new cupcake company, but both of those endeavors had to be put on hold permanently, and she is presently without a job.

"It's really difficult to deal with because I don't know if I will ever feel normal again. It really hits you emotionally as you just want to get better, and I always worry about another relapse because I often think to myself, 'I can't do this again.'" I just don't feel myself while living with this relentless condition.

"I'm not usually very open about my emotions, even to myself, but COVID exploded something inside me so my normal coping mechanisms weren't going to work. I sought counseling because I knew something was wrong. I had a really horrible feeling all the time, like I was reliving the agony of when I was sick. The counseling is helping." The counselor uses various exercises to help me identify my feelings and how I relate to them, like asking me to describe the feeling as a color.

"I use video chats to keep up with my pals, but I need to make sure I'm rested and have the stamina to do so. Talking to others on the Long COVID Facebook Group has been incredibly beneficial, apart from that. It's wonderful to exchange thoughts and speak with folks who really get what you're going through. For this reason, I have created a private Facebook group where we get together on a regular basis to discuss anything from life to symptoms to future goals. I wanted everyone to feel like they're not alone since I understood that some individuals would be having a hard time coping. We support one another in a manner that our friends and family may not be able to.

"Yin yoga, meditation, keeping a mood journal, and creative writing are other activities I've been doing for my own mental health, though I've had to write with my right hand because my left arm doesn't seem to be working."

In December 2021, more than 1.3 million people in the UK—one in fifty of us—were suffering from the symptoms of long-term COVID-19, which include shortness of breath, coughing, chest pain, chronic fatigue, muscle pain, loss of appetite, changes in taste and smell, confusion, depression, and anxiety, according to ONS data.

The Real Story of Extended COVID
Long COVID, also known as Post-Acute Sequelae of SARS-CoV-2 infection (PASC), is a medical challenge that quietly surfaced as the initial waves of the COVID-19 pandemic subsided. Long COVID is a term that describes a variety of symptoms that continue for weeks or even months after the acute phase of the infection has ended. These lingering effects have prompted both scientific investigation and public debate, with some arguing that Long COVID is exaggerated or misrepresented.

Long COVID: What Is It?

Long COVID is a complicated, multi-system illness with a broad range of symptoms, not a single disease. These symptoms might include:

Chronic exhaustion and fogginess

Breathlessness and chest discomfort

Joint and muscle discomfort

Depression, anxiety, and irregular sleep patterns

Palpitations in the heart, lightheadedness, and digestive issues

These symptoms are not limited to persons who had severe COVID-19; they may also affect people who were previously healthy. Some people recover in a few weeks, while others suffer for months, often being unable to return to their regular activities or employment.

Recognition and Scientific Proof

Leading health organizations, such as the World Health Organization (WHO), the U.S. Centers for Disease Control and Prevention (CDC), and the National Institutes of Health (NIH), have acknowledged Long COVID despite early skepticism. Several peer-reviewed studies have verified its existence and documented its effects across a range of populations, irrespective of age or pre-existing medical conditions.

Claims that Long COVID is uncommon or a myth are refuted by large-scale studies, such as the UK Office for National Statistics and the U.S. RECOVER Initiative, which have followed millions of COVID-19 survivors and shown that 10–30% of them have long-term symptoms.

Disputations and False Information

While stress and anxiety can undoubtedly affect health, dismissing Long COVID as hysteria undermines the lived experience of millions and impedes medical advancement. Like much of the

COVID-19 narrative, Long COVID has become a battleground for misinformation. Some fringe voices claim it's a psychological condition, a result of fear and media influence, while others blame it on lockdowns, vaccines, or even mask usage.

Science moves with data, not headlines. The persistence of symptoms after viral infection is not specific to COVID-19; conditions like chronic fatigue syndrome (ME/CFS) and post-viral syndromes have long been recognized after viruses like Epstein-Barr or SARS-1. Additionally, misreporting in the media—sometimes sensationalizing symptoms without scientific backing—has fueled skepticism.

Continued Investigations and Interventions

Investigations into the causes of Long COVID are ongoing, and some theories include:

Overactivation of the immune system

Persistence of viruses in tissues

Blood flow is affected by microclots.

Dysautonomia, or dysfunction of the autonomic nerve system

Research efforts are growing, with clinical studies investigating antivirals, anti-inflammatories, and rehabilitation techniques. Understanding these pathways is essential to creating successful therapies.

While there is currently no cure, targeted treatments, physical therapy, and cognitive rehabilitation have showed promise, and Long COVID clinics have been set up in various countries to assist individuals manage their symptoms.

In order to really transcend the deceptions of the COVID-19 age, we need to be prepared to face harsh realities, particularly when they impact the weak and disregarded. Long COVID necessitates ongoing study, open communication, and most importantly, empathy for individuals dealing with its difficulties.

Five to ten percent of COVID patients have long-lasting symptoms that persist three months or more.

Several biological processes have been postulated by researchers to explain long COVID. However, in a perspective piece published in the most recent issue of the Medical Journal of Australia, we contend that the persistence of the virus in the body seems to be the primary cause of most, if not all, of long COVID.

A concept known as "viral persistence" has been recognized from the beginning of the pandemic: in some individuals, SARS-CoV-2, or at least fragments of the virus, may remain in different tissues and organs for prolonged periods of time.

Although it is now generally known that some people's bodies retain residual viral pieces for an extended period of time, it is less clear if active virus, rather than just old virus fragments, is still present and whether this is the source of prolonged COVID.

This difference is important because some antiviral strategies may target living viruses in ways that "dead" viral pieces cannot.

There are two important consequences of viral persistence:

When it manifests in some individuals with severe immunocompromised conditions, it is believed to be the cause of novel and significantly dissimilar variations, such JN.1.
Long COVID may be caused by a long-lasting infection, meaning that it may continue to produce symptoms in a large number of persons in the general population long after the acute disease has ended.
What is the conclusion of the research?

Even while there isn't yet a single research that proves a persistent virus causes prolonged COVID, a number of recent important publications together provide a strong argument. Many persons with moderate COVID symptoms had prolonged periods of shedding the virus's genetic material, known as viral RNA, from their respiratory system, according to a February research published in Nature.

Long-term COVID was more likely to affect those who had consistent shedding of this viral RNA, which most likely indicates the existence of live virus.

reproducing viral RNA and proteins were found in patient blood fluid years after the original infection by other important studies. This suggests that the virus is probably reproducing for extended periods of time in some secret reservoirs inside the body, maybe including blood cells.

Another research indicated that individuals with consistently positive viral RNA had a greater risk of protracted COVID (measured four months after infection), and that viral RNA was discovered in ten distinct tissue locations and blood samples 1–4 months after acute infection.

The gastrointestinal system is one area of significant interest as a long-term viral hideaway, and the same research provided hints regarding the location of the persistent virus.

In the RECOVER initiative, a joint research endeavor that strives to address the implications of long COVID, more evidence of a persistent virus boosting the chance of long COVID was reported earlier this week.

However, since it is technically difficult to isolate the live virus from reservoirs within the body where the virus "hides," official evidence that a virus capable of reproducing may persist in the body for years is still elusive.

Without it, experts like us contend that the body of evidence is now strong enough to spur action.

What must occur next?

Accelerated testing of established antivirals for the prevention and treatment of chronic COVID is the logical solution to this.

In the case of long-term COVID, this should include more unconventional treatments, including the diabetic medication metformin, which may have two advantages:

its antiviral qualities, which have shown unexpected effectiveness against protracted COVID

as a viable treatment for fatigue-related deficits. However, the creation of clinical trial platforms for quick testing and the development of novel medications should be another top priority.

Exciting treatment possibilities have been discovered by science, but converting them into forms that can be used in clinical settings is a significant challenge that calls for government funding and assistance.

What leads to prolonged COVID?

Why some persons have a prolonged COVID while others recover a few weeks after infection is yet unknown.

It would provide us with hints if it were merely associated with severe COVID, but it isn't since we have seen individuals in critical care who have long-lasting COVID symptoms.

Nonetheless, several innovative concepts have been proposed by scholars worldwide.

This includes the theory that prolonged COVID may result from people's immune systems malfunctioning and overworking after infection.

It is possible that the vaccine could help by rerouting the immune system back on track, by directly activating certain immune cells like T cells (which help stimulate antibody production and kill virus-infected cells) or frontline innate immune cells that correct this immune misfiring. One clue that supports this theory is that some people with long COVID report that their symptoms significantly improve after receiving a COVID vaccine. This strongly suggests the various symptoms of long COVID are directly linked back to our immune system.

According to another theory, individuals with long-lasting COVID may have a small, persistent "viral reservoir" in their bodies that is undetectable by diagnostic tests, or small, unresolved viral fragments that are not contagious but may regularly trigger the immune system. A vaccine may help target the immune system to the appropriate locations in order to eliminate the remaining virus.

Although we cannot yet be certain that a vaccination would benefit everyone, there is no proof that suppressing the immune system worsens the situation; on the contrary, it is probably going to improve it.

In the long run, COVID may be a mix of these two factors or a variety of other factors.

In the end, we still need more research since it is still in its early phases. Although there is currently no treatment, we can help people with their symptoms and urge everyone to receive the COVID-19 vaccination when it becomes available.

Made in the USA
Monee, IL
28 July 2025